ALL ABOUT DEPRESSION

ADD COLORS TO YOUR LIFE

DIPTESH GHOSH

THIS BOOK IS DEDICATED WITH LOVE AND AFFECTION TO

MY FATHER LATE DINESH CH.GHOSH

AND TO ALL

MY FAMILY MEMBERS

Contents

1. Depression   1

2. Depression Different From Sadness   2

3. Cause Of Depression   4

4. Types Of Depression   6

5. Depression Symptoms Vary With Gender And Age   12

6. Symptoms Of Depression   15

7. Methods To Keep Depression Away   16

8. Diet Related To Depression   20

Foods That Helps To Fight Depression

Foods That Can Cause Depression

9. Conclusion   25

ONE

DEPRESSION

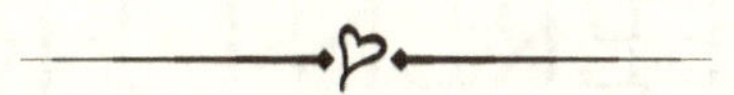

The word depression often mis-understood and used as a synonym for sadness. It is the normal human reaction to denote low mood or feeling sad as depression. Nevertheless, depression is more than just a low mood. It is a serious mental illness that negatively affects how we feel, think and act in our daily activities. In fact, depression is a devastating illness has turned into a global epidemic. Most interestingly, the rate of depression is increasing from generation after generation. However, depression is a condition that affects us physically and mentally. Some of us experience these feelings intensely, for a long period may be for a week, months or even years and with no apparent reason. Depression is a negative mental state of mind. Fortunately, it is treatable. Those who are in a depressed state of mind experience a prolonged feeling of sadness and hopelessness and does not find interest in any of the activities they have once enjoyed. However, if depression left untreated for a long period it may turn into a serious health problem. There are many positive methods through which we can uplift our mood to overcome depression and regain the beauty of life.

TWO

DEPRESSION DIFFERENT FROM SADNESS

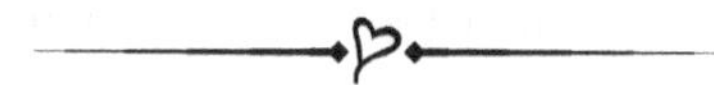

The most significant symptom connected with depression is sadness but it is hard to make a difference between the two psychological states of mind.

However, depression is a step ahead of just sadness, and not simply by a measure of degree. The difference between these two states of mind is not to what extent a person feels down, but a combination of factors like duration of these negative feelings, other symptoms, bodily impact, and the effect upon the individual's capability to work in daily life.

Sadness is an emotion that each one of us will experience in our lifetime. It may be the loss of a job, or end of a relationship, or maybe the death of our closed relatives. Sadness may come from a particular situation, person, or event. In the case of depression, in fact, no such reason is required. Depression makes a man or a woman feels sad or hopeless about everything in their life. They could have made their life much more beautiful and yet they lose the ability to experience joy or pleasure.

In case of sadness, one might feel down in the dumps for a day or two, but they still can enjoy simple things like their favorite TV show, food, or spending time with friends. This might not be the case when someone is dealing with depression. The same activities from which once they had enjoyed are no longer interesting or pleasurable to them.

When one feels sadness for a certain incident or reason, he or she will be able to sleep as usual and can do things to motivate themselves as well as maintain their desire to eat. On the other hand, who is going through depression will lose his or her normal food intake. Their sleeping patterns will also change either not wanting to get out of bed all day or may be suffering from insomnia.

The basic difference in these two states of mind is their way of thinking. Sad people might feel regret or repent for the activities they did, but they won't feel any permanent sense of worthlessness or guilt as in case of a depressed person. Self-diminishing is another negative thought patterns commonly found symptoms among the depressed

Finally, self-harm and suicidal thought does not come from non-depressive sadness. Thoughts of self-harm, death, or suicide, or have a suicide plan are very much common among severely depressed persons.

In spite of the fact that there is a clear distinction between depression and sadness, there are chances for the major depressive disorder to occur from prolonged sadness resulting from grief financial loss or a serious medical illness.

THREE
CAUSE OF DEPRESSION

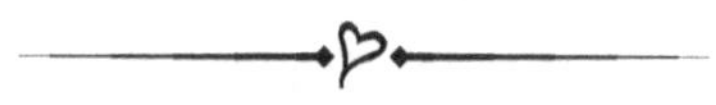

The exact cause of depression has not yet been pinpointed as a number of things are often related to the development of depression. A single issue or recent event is not responsible for depression, as it may be a combination of recent events and other longer-term or personal factors. In today's world of 7.7 billion (aug 2019) populations, we might have millions of reasons toget depressed. The triggerscannot be generalized as every single individual gets depressed for different reasons but researchers have found a common fundamental primary trigger that is the brain's runaway stress response commonly known as a stress response. Here are some of the reasons for which one might get depressed but there may be many other reasons depend upon the individual's situation.

Life events – Observation revealed that continuing difficulties like long-term unemployment, living in an obnoxious relationship, long-term isolation, and prolonged work stress – are some of the reasons why we get depressed. The passing away of a family member, friend, or pets can lead to depression as it goes beyond normal grief. The divorce of parents, their separation, or remarry — can be the reason of depression among the children.

One should always keep in mind that whatever the adverse life situations lead to depression, it depends a lot on how well he or she can handle the situation by staying positive.

Family history – An Individual having Depression history within his or her family members will be at high genetic risk of depression. However, having a genetic history of depression does not mean you will have the same experience. Personal factors and circumstances of the individuals are still likely to have an important role to play. Therefore, genes may be one of the factor, but not the only factor for depression

Personality – An individual having a tendency to get anxious, having low self-confidence, perfectionists, and sensitive to personal criticism, may be more at risk of depression.

Serious medical illness– Anindividual dealing with long-termserious illness, chronic pain may lead to depression. They need very good family support apart from Doctors to bring them out from depression.

Drug and alcohol use– A very interesting observation made regarding drug and alcohol. Too much addiction to Drug and alcohol can lead to depression. On the other hand, many depressed people take the help of drug and alcohol to get out of their problems. This is a very negative approach and not at all recommended

Brain chemistry – Chemicals called neurotransmitters send messages between the nerve cells in the brain. Some of the neurotransmitters regulate mood. When the supplies of neurotransmitters are low or not effective we get depressed. Daylight helps the brain to produces melatonin and serotonin. These neurotransmitters help to regulate the activity of an individual . Less sunlight means more melatonin and eventually less serotonin. This imbalance of neurotransmitters helps to create the conditions for depression known as a seasonal affective disorder (SAD). Exposure to sunlight helps to improve mood for the people affected by SAD. Regular exercise and enough sleep also have a very positive effect on neurotransmitter activity and mood. We still know very little about this chemical imbalance of the brain.

Thyroid disease - When a butterfly-shaped gland in our neck unable to produce enough thyroid hormone (hypothyroidism) the symptom of depression arises. The main function of this multifunctional hormone is to act as a neurotransmitter and regulate the level of serotonin. The thyroid test is unavoidable if the symptom of depression comes with cold sensitivity constipation as well as fatigue.

Internet addiction – Various researches revealed that too much time spending on the internet might lead to lack of companionship or real-life interaction with family and friends. This, in turn, takes particularly the teens and preteens to depression. In fact, the researchers are still confused in finding out whether overuse of internet leads to depression or depressed use internet.

FOUR
TYPES OF DEPRESSION

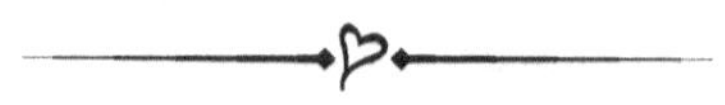

Depression may come in different shapes and forms. In order to get an effective treatment, it is very important to know the types of depression

Major depression– Major depression is also known as major depressive disorder, classic depression, or unipolar depression. Major depression is fairly a common type of depression which people experience symptoms most of the day, every day. Major depression is not related to what is happening around us. In spite of having all positive situations, we might still have depression.

The symptoms of this severe depression may be-

- Unhappiness, dimness, or grief
- Insomnia or too much sleep
- Lack of liveliness and tiredness
- Loss of appetite or overeating
- Aches and pains with no proper medical explanation.
- Lack of interest in pleasurable activities
- Lack of self-application, short memory, and lack of ability to make decisions
- Feelings of worthlessness or hopelessness
- Constant worry and nervousness
- Thoughts of death, self-harm, or suicide

Symptoms can last for weeks or even months. Some people might experience a single episode of major depression, while others experience it throughout their life. Major depression creates problems in our relationships and daily life.

Persistent depression– Persistent depressive disorder is a form of depression that can last for a year or more. It's also known as Dysthymia or chronic depression. The intensity of this type of depression is low in comparison with major depression but still can create problems in our relationships and daily life.

The symptoms of this persistent depression may be-

- Deep sadness or hopelessness.
- Lack of self-confidence or feelings of inadequacy.
- Lack of interest in a pleasant activity.
- Change in appetite.
- Change in sleeping patterns and low energy.
- Lack of attention and a short memory.
- Difficulty functioning at school or work
- Inability to feel joy, even on happy occasions
- Social withdrawal

In spite of the fact that it is a long-term type of depression, the severity level does not remain the same throughout the period. The level of intensity of symptoms goes up and down. As the persistent depression runs for a long time the suffer starts feeling the symptoms as a part of their life. Some major depression symptoms are noticed while having a persistent depressive disorder, which is termed as double depression.

Manic depression or bipolar disorder– One experiences alternating spells of depression happiness in manic depression. Depression obsession is the old name of the bipolar disorder. To diagnose bipolar disorder, one should experience an episode of mania that lasts seven days; one may experience a depressive episode before or after the manic episode.

Depressive depression may have the same symptoms like major depression, including:

- Feelings of sadness and emptiness.
- Lack of energy.
- Fatigue
- Sleep problems
- Trouble concentrating
- Decreased activity
- Loss of interest in formerly enjoyable activities

- Suicidal thought.

Signs of a manic phase include.

- High energy
- Reduced sleep
- Bad temper
- Racing thoughts and speech, excessive thinking
- Increased self-esteem and confidence
- Unusual, risky, and self-destructive behavior
- Feeling elate "high," or excited

In severe cases, episodes can include hallucinations and delusions. Hypomania is a less severe form of mania. We can also have mixed episodes where we have symptoms of both mania and depression.

Depressive psychosis– Some people with major depression experience periods of loss of contact with reality. This is termed as psychosis, which can lead to hallucinations and disappointments. The experience of these two aspects clinically termed as a major depressive disorder with psychotic characteristics. However, some refer to this phenomenon as depressive psychosis or psychotic depression. Hallucinations are, when you see, hear, smell, taste or feel things that do not really exist. An example of this would be hearing voices or seeing people who are not present. Delirium is a strongly held belief that is clearly false or meaningless. But for someone who is experiencing psychosis, all these things are very real and true. Depression with psychosis can also cause physical symptoms, including problems with constant or slow physical movements.

Perinatal depression–Perinatal depression is clinically known as a major depressive disorder with peripartum initiation occurs during pregnancy or within four weeks after delivery. It is also known as postpartum depression. However, this term only applies to postpartum depression. Perinatal depression can occur during pregnancy.

The hormonal changes that occur during pregnancy and childbirth can trigger changes in the brain that lead to mood swings. Not even the lack of sleep and physical discomfort that often accompany pregnancy and the fact of having a newborn.

Symptoms of perinatal depression may include:

- Sadness
- Anxiety
- Anger or rage
- Exhaustion
- Extreme worry about the baby's health and safety
- The problem in self-caring as well as for the new baby
- Thoughts of self-harm or harming the baby

Those women lacking family support or having a history of previous depression episode are at increased risk of developing perinatal depression but can happen to anyone.

Premenstrual dysphoric disorder or PMDD is a serious form of premenstrual syndrome (PMS). While the symptoms of premenstrual syndrome can be both physical and psychological, the symptoms of PMDD tend to be mostly psychological.

These psychological symptoms are more severe than those associated with premenstrual syndrome are. For example, some women may feel more emotional in the days leading up to their period. However, someone with PMDD may experience a level of depression and sadness that interferes with daily functions.

Other possible symptoms of PMDD include:

- Cramp, swell and breast tenderness.
- A headache, joint and muscle pain.
- Sadness, feel despair.
- Irritability and anger extreme mood swings.
- Less desire to eat or overeat.
- Panic or anxiety attacks.
- Lack of energy and problems to concentrate
- Irregular sleep.

Similar to perinatal depression PMDD is also related to hormonal changes. The symptoms often begin immediately after ovulation and begin to fade once you have the cycle.Some women reject PMDD as a serious case of PMS, but PMDD can become very serious and include thoughts of suicide

Seasonal depression, also called seasonal affective disorder and clinically known as a major depressive disorder with a seasonal pattern, is related to certain seasons, mainly during the winter months.

Symptoms often begin in the fall of winter, as the days begin to shrink and continue throughout the winter. They include:

- Social retirement.
- Greater need to sleep.
- Weight gain.
- Everyday feelings of sadness, despair or indignity.

Seasonal depression may worsen as the season progresses and lead to suicidal thoughts. Once spring begins, the symptoms tend to improve. This could be related to changes in body rhythms in response to the increase in natural light.

Situational depression, clinically known as an adjustment disorder with a depressed mood, appears to be a major depression in many aspects.
But it is caused by specific events or situations, such as:

- The death of a loved one serious illness or another potentially lethal event.
- Pass for divorce or custody of children.
- Be in emotional or physically violent relationships.
- Being unemployed or facing serious financial difficulties.
- Face serious legal problems.

Of course, it is normal to feel sad and anxious during events like these, even to retire for a while from others. But situational depression occurs when these feelings begin to feel disproportionate to the triggering event and interfere with your daily life.
The symptoms of situational depression tend to begin within three months of the initial event and may include:

- Frequent crying.
- Sadness and despair.
- Anxiety.
- Changes in appetite.
- Difficulty to sleep.
- Aches and pains.
- Lack of energy and fatigue.

- Inability to concentrate.
- Social retirement.

FIVE

DEPRESSION SYMPTOMS VARY WITH GENDER AND AGE

The symptoms of depression differ from person to person as well as from one age group to another. The symptoms may also vary from gender to gender. There are several common symptoms for each age group with common triggers

Depression in men

Depressed men do not show the signs of self-hatred and hopelessness rather they complain about their tiredness, shows bad temper, have sleeping problems and less concentration in their work and hobbies. Symptoms like anger, aggression and reckless behavior are common in depressed men.

Depression in women

Women experience depression symptoms like prominent feelings of guilt, oversleeping or overeating resulting in weight gain. Depression in women is the result of imbalance hormonal factors during menstruation, pregnancy, and menopause. Every 1 woman out of 7 experience depression after childbirth.

Children 0- 12 years

Depressions among the children below 12 years are not very common. But sometimes depression is noticed as they could not express themselves very clearly to the world. Often it is found that as they could not cope up with the new situation in school, learning problem, new friends or loss of interest in entertaining activities they feel sad or hopeless resulting weight gain or loss, anxiety and lethargy.Parents in these cases should take the help of pediatrician as well as counselor. This should not be left uncared for a long time as the normal development of the child may hamper.

Teens 12 – 18 years

This is an age when we are exposed every day to a new world with different situations. Teens always have some dreams of fantasy in their mind. It happens sometimes that they could not match their dreams with their real life and thus having problems in schools with parents and friends and so on. Depression in teens may also crop up from pressures to fit in, be successful, hormonal issues or by any types of rejection. This changes their moods, which may last longer than a few weeks. These issues can lead young children's to depression resulting to an extent of self-harm behavior or alcohol and drug use.

Symptoms are like unusual levels of irritations; feelings of worthlessness, fits of anger often noticed. Depressed teens do not show sign of sadness. They always complain of headaches, stomachaches, or other physical pains.Too much sleeping eating avoiding friends and others or less participation in activities are also some of the symptoms.

The suspected depressed teens are to be dealt with a very sensitive manner. In order to fill confidence and reduce their pressure, parents should interact with them in a positive manner. Doctor's advice is also important to determine whether the symptoms are due to physical imbalances like hypothyroidism. Counseling by a mental health professional is also very helpful and highly recommended.

Young Adults19 – 29

This is the major transition period of life where different situations can lead to depression. Financial instability, not coping up with office environment or relationship issues are some of the common reasons which can lead to depression. One should have a very good support system of family members, friends, and therapist to guide through this transition period of life and get them out of depression.

Midlife Adults30 – 60

Adults within the age group of 30 to 60 have a lot of reasons that can activate depression. Some of them may be responsibilities of family, financial stress, work and relationship issues, menopause, or major illnesses. Depression among the women under this age group is common. Apart from regular signs of depression, some might exhibit anger, rude or violent behavior. Encouragement or listening to their concern helps them to get out of depression. Primary care from doctors is helpful, who can assess if any medication or physical issues involved in their problem.

Senior Adults 61+

Depression is common among the senior adults but the most tragic part is that they are often overlooked or left untreated. Seniors adults may develop depression from late-life issues, isolation, and death of a spouse. Financial constraints, Illnesses and the use of unnecessary medicine can also lead to depression. Symptoms in seniors includes insomnia, weakness, sadness, and anxiety, short memory physical aches and pains.

In fact, our society has a great role to play in eradicating the depression among the senior adults. We should always show love and respect for them. We should give them companion so that they do not feel lonely or isolated. Periodical family gathering or outing with family yields a great result. In any case, we should follow doctor's advice as treatment can help to get rid of their depression.

SIX

SYMPTOMS OF DEPRESSION

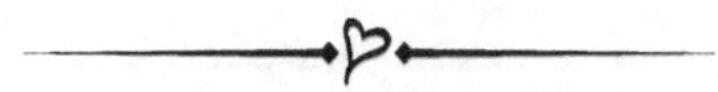

The common signs and symptoms of depression vary from individual to individual, gender to gender and from age group to group. It actually depends on the individual's situation. But most importantly it should be kept in mind that all these symptoms are part of our normal life in low key. But if these signs and symptoms are stronger in terms of behavior and stay longer that means the person is dealing with depression. Some common symptoms of depression may be

1. Helpless and worthless feeling, sad tearfulness, or emptiness along with guilty feeling on past failures or self-blaming.

2. Loss of interest in daily normal activities like sex, hobbies, cooking or sports.

3. Change in appetite which results in either weight gain or weight loss.

4. Insomnia or too much sleeping.

5. Showing anger, irritation or frustration even over small matters. Nervousness, agitation or restlessness is also some of the noticeable behaviors.

6. Energy Loss or tiredness resulting work phobia.

7. Self-hatred, thoughts of death and suicide.

8. Irresponsible or thoughtless behavior as well as trouble in taking a decision.

9. Short memory, lack of concentration.

10. Feeling of physical problems like back pain or headaches aches with no proper medical explanation.

11. Slowness in thought, dialogue or body activities.

SEVEN

METHODS TO KEEP DEPRESSION AWAY

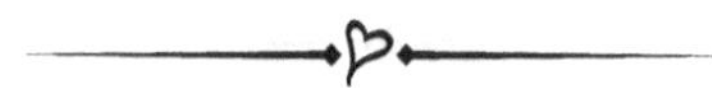

Every one of us should do our best to keep ourselves mentally stable and be a positive person. Mental well-being is one of the most underestimated problems that everyone should take care of above everything else. The most tragic part of the modern age disease called depression is that we do not even realize that we are the victims of depression. Thus, it is better to take some preventive measures before we get depressed.

As depression is a serious mentalillness that negatively affects how we feel, think and act, we should always try to boost up our mental condition with positive thoughts. It is the natural phenomenon that days are followed by night. That means bad patches of life are followed by good time. Keep calm during the bad patches of life and think of the happy moments of the past. Everything will be on the right path again. If we cannot laugh, over and again on the same joke then there is no point in crying over and again on the same problem and in the process making ourselves depressed. There are some techniques following which we can keep depression away.

1. Personal diary - Writing is a form of treatment that we should make a habit every day. To be honest, it is difficult to open ourselves up and talk about our feelings with the society. It is as because sometimes the reactions of the people are extremely critical. Thus in order to express what is going on inside we should take a few minutes out of our daily routine to write it down. There is no fixed format. It can be our realization or moments of sadness, anxiousness or even happiness. We can write down five things that we love about ourselves, five things that we want to improve on, and what we can do to change in our life. Initially, it will not be easy to express oneself in a piece of paper but once it becomes a practice, it will give great mental relief.

2. Love your life – Our life is short and therefore we should give every priority to make it lively and happy. In order to make our life happy we need to love our life and do accordingly what our hearts say. We should eat delicious food (unless it is harmful to health), take a walk, have fun, watch favorite T.V programs and do whatever that lights up our heart. We should find our passion, which will make us feel alive.

3. Talk to someone – Sometimes writing down as motioned earlier is not enough. Then we need to talk to someone in order to release our negativity. The person whom we chose may be a therapist, a close friend or a relative. However, it is important to keep in mind that the person whom we choose should be willing to hear our problems with positive notes.

4. Speak well of yourself – We are not always perfect as we are human beings. We all have bad moments and do mistakes in our life. Nevertheless, we should not highlight those mistakes instead talk to ourselves that we are human beings and can rectify our mistakes. On the other hand, if we highlight our own mistakes, there are people who will laugh at us and make us feel bad about our self. And the result is often getting into depression.

5. Set a routine for your goal –In today's busy worldweshouldalways structure our daily life with daily goals. Setting a daily schedule can help us to complete our task within a period and can give a feeling of achieving something. This feeling of achievement will boost up our energy to go for the next project or work. Initially setting small goals or targets means the more chances of achievement, which in turn will boost our confidence to achieve big targets of our life. And the achievements keeps the depression away.

6. Step out into the sunlight – Expose to sunlight helps to release serotonin and endorphins that lead to a happier mood. It keeps our bones healthy by producing vitamin D and absorbs calcium. Thus sunlight has a positive effect on the mental and physical status of our health. Therefore, regular exposing to sunlight should be our habit.

7. Laugh – This five-letter word can really change our world. A smile can increase our face value to a great extent and ease the tension of our muscles. Laughing helps the brain to release chemicals that fight pain and infections. Therefore we should wake up every morning with a smile. If we have no reason to smile then at least we can think of some happy moments, which will make us happy. It should be our regular practice. Smiling will not only make us happy but will also create a positive environment.

8. Eat a healthy and balanced diet – Thereis no magical diet, which can keep depression away. As depression tends to overeat, controlled food intake will make us feel better. Our daily diet must include 1,500mg of omega-3 in the form of fish oil capsules, with multi-vitamin and 500mg vitamin C. Omega-3 fatty acids like salmon and tuna and folic acids like spinach and avocado could help to ease depression. Briefly, a balanced diet means as high in omega-3 fat, healthy fats and a moderate amount of animal protein.

9. Enough sleep – Our human body including brain is designed in such a way that too much or too little sleep can create problem in the total system. We need eight hours of full sound sleep. Try to avoid now and then napping. It is important to maintain the same time to go and get out of bed regularly. Another important point to be kept in mind is that we should keep ourselves away from all electronic gadgets like mobile, T.V. etc at least an hour before we go to bed. These small changes in lifestyle can improve our sleeping habits.

10. Exercise – If we look back to our ancestors, we will find that they were not as depressed as we are today. It is because they were engaged in more physical work than we are in today's life. Their mode of lifestyle was different from today's modern lifestyle. They were engaged in vigorous physical activities like hunting, agriculture, fishing and so on. In the process, biologically they produced more BDNF Gene a compound that helps to increase the production of new neurons and neuronal connectivity. Thus, regular exercise can encourage the brain to rewire itself in positive ways. We cannot virtually do any exercise in our today's busy schedule and that makes the difference. However, if we can develop a habit of at least 30 minutes of fast walking every alternate day it will give a better result than the drugs with a side effect.

11. Meditation - During the depression the brain works in crisis management. Therefore the first and foremost thing to do during depression is to keep calm. And calmness of mind is possible only through meditation. From medical point of view it has been found that during depression the medical prefrontal cortex region of brain gets hyperactive. As a result we start worrying about our future and have the same thoughts of past again and again. Another region of brain called amygdale is responsible for fight-or-flight response. It helps to release stress hormone(cortisol) from adrenal glands resulting to activate fear response. These two regions of our brain works off each other and cause depression. Meditation breaks the connection between these two regions and thus helps to reduce depression.

Researchers have found that a depressed brain has smaller volume of grey matter in their hippocampus. A regular meditation helps to increase the volume of grey matter as well as protects the hippocampus and there by improves our memory.

A short meditation of five to ten minutes every morning and night helps to lead a positive and depression free life.

12. Doing something new – Always incorporate a new lifestyle in your life in order to avoid the daily monotony of life. A monotonous life can take us to aRuminative state of mind and ultimately lead to depression. We should push our self to do something new like going to a new place, learning a new language or a musical instrument and so on. This activity of doing something new will change the levels of our brain chemical like dopamine which trigger up our pleasure and enjoyment. In a nut shell it can be said that we should be always busy with new positive works and thoughts to get a depression free life.

13. Social Connection – If we focus back in the history of mankind we will find that we have survived in this planet earth through living in groups. Through ages we have develop a mental frame of mind to live and work in a group format. But now a days due to our fast pace of life we are getting away from each other mentally. We might have thousands of facebook friends but with no real close friends with whom we can spend our time. As our brain is not designed for isolation and produce hormones. We need face to face interaction for proper functioning of brain. Thus we should convert social media to social occasion to keep depression away.

14. Will power – Will power is perhaps the most important tool to fight against depression. If we can create a strong will rather fill confidence within ourselves nothing in the world can pour us into depression. Building confidence within us is a continuous process and we should always talk to ourselves with positive notes.

EIGHT

DIET RELATED TO DEPRESSION

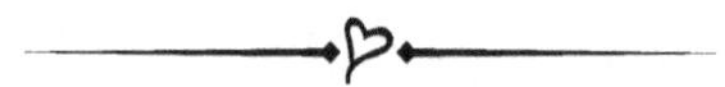

Diet related to depression can be divided into two categories. One is the foods that help to fight depression away and the other is the food that is detrimental for depression. But it will be fair enough to give a statutory warning that before fixing up any diet we must consult the physician. It is because for example an egg is good for fighting depression as it contains protein and zinc. But eggs are not at all advisable for those who are having kidney problems or having allergic reactions.

Foods that helps to fight depression

It has been proved that, if the below mentioned foods are added in our diet it will help us to fight depression

1. Green tea – Green teacontain many antioxidants and L-theanine, amino acids that help us to fight depression. Green tea contains amino acid which increases the level of dopamine and there by decrease the level of stress and anxiety. Three to four cups daily will help to uplift our mood. Nuts, whole grains, broccoli also contains L-theanine.

2. Almonds –Almonds containa lot of magnesium which helps to make serotonin. Low level of magnesium in the body will show the signs of depression as well as less energetic.100 gram of almonds have more or less about 268 milligrams of magnesium Therefore inclusion of almonds in our daily diet will keep us active and depression free throughout the day.

3.Omega3 – Omega6 and omega3 play a complementary role in our body. Omega6 is inflammatory and omega3 is anti-inflammatory. Our body is designed to have a balance of omega6 & omega3 in a ratio of 1:1. The optimal tolerable ratio is can 3:1. But due to modern day fast and processed food this ratio has gone up to 17:1 and lead to depression. So we need to supplement omega3 through our diets. Foods like roasted soya beans, walnuts,salmon sardine & mackerel fish, Canola Oil, Chia Seeds, flaxseeds contains high amount of omega 3. Regular inclusion of these foods yields a good result for anti depression.

4. Dark chocolate – Darkchocolatesacts as anti depressants because it increases the level of serotonin. Dark chocolate slows down the production of stress hormones which lessen anxiety and chronic fatigue syndrome. One ounces of dark chocolate daily is the right dose for depression.

5. Eggs – Eggs are full of protein and other Nutrients like zinc. Zinc is needed by our body to produce neurotransmitters. Eggs also contain vitamin D lack of which is related to depression and mental health problems.

6. Bananas - Bananas contain tryptophan which increases the body's serotonin level. Tyrosine is also required for making nor epinephrine and dopamine the two important neurotransmitters that boost up our mood. Thus one or two bananas daily will help us to get out of depression or low mood. Other high sources of tryptophan are turkey, crab watercress etc.

7. Avocados - Avocados contains a great amount of omega-3 fatty acids that helps to move serotonin a neurotransmitter that is responsible for the feelings of happiness. 100 grams of avocado contains 485 milligrams of potassium, and an adult needs about 4500 to 4700 milligrams of potassium daily. Avocados are also full of amino acid (tryptophan) that helps to reduce stress and relax.

8. Blueberries - Blueberries contains the highest antioxidant capacity among the popular fruits and vegetables. The antioxidants help our brain to function properly and delay our mental depression. It also contains vitamin B complex and selenium zinc potassium that keeps our brain healthy.

9. Spinach - Spinach is filled with nutrients like folic acid magnesium and zinc which helps the brain to remain healthy and fight depression. It also contains several other vitamins and minerals among which particularly vitamin B plays an important role in enzyme production.

10. Asparagus – This green veggie is reach in vitamin B12and folic acid apart from many other nutrients. Proper amount of B12 and folic acid is very important for neurological function. Getting some asparagus in our daily diet can be helpful to fight depression.

Foods that can cause depression

Many researches revealed that choice of food makes the difference between feeling good or worse. Thus we need to reduce the consumption of those foods that are linked to cause anxiety and depression. Some of them are as follows.

1. Sugar – It is one of the most addicted item that every one of us love to take. When we intake sugar the blood glucose levels are elevated and the levels of protein that helps the growth of neurons and synapses drops. The recommended amount of daily sugar intake for adult women 25 grams and adult men 36 grams

2. Artificial Sweeteners – Aspartame is an artificial sweetener used in some food and beverages. But the bad side of aspartame is that it obstructs the production of the neurotransmitter serotonin resulting insomnia, mood change.

3. Alcohol – Consumption of alcohol hampers the function of our central nervous system. Our central nervous system takes the information through the senses, controlling motor function, as well as thinking, understanding, and reasoning. It also controls emotion. Alcohol slows all this down, aggravate symptoms associated with depression. We should limit our alcohol consumption to a glass or two of red wine a week. Try gluten-free alcohol. The best thing may be to go alcohol-free and relax with some probiotic-rich, fermented cold drinks.

4. Processed food– Intake too much of refined or processed carbohydrates — like white bread, cereal, pasta, or snacks may cause the same impact on our blood sugar levels as eating a container of jelly beans After the initial dose insulin we will find ourselves exhausted irritated, and depressed.

5. Hydrogenated oils–Any food that is cooked with hydrogenated oils and contains trans-fats (unsaturated fats) can contribute depression. Thus it better to stay away from the fried chicken, the fried cheese sticks, fried calamari, and French fries. Saturated fats found in animal products like deli meats, high-fat dairy, butter, etc. can block arteries and stop blood flow to the brain and there by hampers the optimal brain function.

6. Foods high in sodium– There is a general conception among us that the solution for weight loss is to take fat free food. But these fat-free foods contains high amount of sodium that disrupt our neurological system, contributing to depression. It can also mess up our immune system response, resulting fatigue. Excess salt consumption leads to fluid retention and bloating.

7. Caffeine– Studies revealed that there is higher percentage of depression among the coffee drinkers. The reason behind it may be coffee disrupts sleep, making it more difficult to fall asleep and to stay asleep. And we all know that Sleep is connected to mood and disturbed sleep can seriously mess with our mental state. The caffeine found in coffee change our mood by impacting hormones, neurotransmitter function and nerve signaling, all things that can leave you feeling less than stellar. It also increases our heart beat rate and makes us more anxious. If we get coffee addict, then without it can lead us to withdrawal symptoms like headaches, drowsiness and a lack of energy. The best alternative may be green tea which is not only anti-aging but contain less caffeine than coffee.

NINE
CONCLUSION

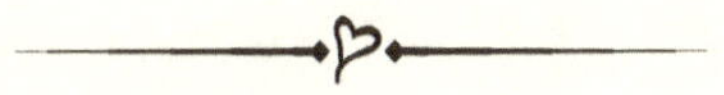

Finally because depression is strongly linked to excess morbidity and mortality, it cannot be left untreated only by primary care doctors. Patients who suffer from diabetes, ischemic heart disease, stroke, or lung disorders that have concurrent depression have poorer outcomes than those without depression. Fifteen percent of patients with severe mood disorders die from suicide. Having said all these I would like to say that don't take life so serious. As every information is limited my views may not match with others and vice versa. And here starts the conflicts and the brain starts all sorts of negative thinking. Thus we should prepare our thoughts in such a way that may be yes may be our opponent is right. This small word "may be" ends all conflicts and we will be able to sustain positive thoughts in ourselves. We should focus our thoughts based on reality rather than on believe.

Another important way to get rid of depression is contentment. We should always be content with whatever little we have got. This will create a heart full of gratitude, thankfulness towards the society and we will be relaxed. It will also help us to cut off our ego and sustain positive thoughts for long and lead a depression free life. It is no mistake that after going through **ALL ABOUT DEPRESSION** if we can make a little bit of addition and alteration in our life we will surely be able to add colours in our life.

The End

www.ingramcontent.com/pod-product-compliance
Lightning Source LLC
Chambersburg PA
CBHW051428250726
48655CB00003B/1291